DAWN KASHUBA

Nutrition for Beginners Simplified

A Comprehensive 10-Step Guide to Mastering Macros, Embracing Real Food, and Selecting Recommended Supplements

Copyright © 2024 by Dawn Kashuba

All rights reserved. No part of this publication may be reproduced, stored or transmitted in any form or by any means, electronic, mechanical, photocopying, recording, scanning, or otherwise without written permission from the publisher. It is illegal to copy this book, post it to a website, or distribute it by any other means without permission.

Dawn Kashuba asserts the moral right to be identified as the author of this work.

Dawn Kashuba has no responsibility for the persistence or accuracy of URLs for external or third-party Internet Websites referred to in this publication and does not guarantee that any content on such Websites is, or will remain, accurate or appropriate.

Designations used by companies to distinguish their products are often claimed as trademarks. All brand names and product names used in this book and on its cover are trade names, service marks, trademarks and registered trademarks of their respective owners. The publishers and the book are not associated with any product or vendor mentioned in this book. None of the companies referenced within the book have endorsed the book.

First edition

This book was professionally typeset on Reedsy.
Find out more at reedsy.com

"The Body won't Go where the mind won't
Let it "

Unknown

Contents

1

Introduction

Introduction

Welcome to the beginning of your journey into understanding the fundamentals of nutrition, which promises to enlighten and empower you with the knowledge to transform your health and lifestyle. This book, "Nutrition for Beginners Simplified," was born from a simple yet profound desire to demystify the complex world of nutritional science and make it accessible to everyone. Whether you're looking to overhaul your diet or simply better understand how food affects your body and mind, you've come to the right place.

The inspiration behind this guide stems from a personal quest for knowledge and the realization that, despite the abundance of information available, there remains a gap between scientific jargon and practical application. My journey into the depths of nutritional science was fueled by curiosity and frustration — curiosity about the intricate dance of nutrients within our bodies and frustration over the myriad of conflicting advice that clouds our path to wellness. I discovered the power of simplicity through navigating this maze of misinformation and complexity. This book is my attempt to share that power with you.

Now, I want to introduce myself and tell you A little about myself: I am a woman in my late 40s who has spent much of my adult life wrestling with the challenge of reclaiming my figure and sense of self after having children. It was a journey that saw me momentarily lose my way, a period during which reaching out for help from medical practitioners often felt like speaking into a void. The responses I received were frequently dismissive, favoring quick-fix prescriptions over genuine, sustainable solutions. This experience left me determined not to settle for inadequate advice and medication as my only recourse.

Fuelled by this determination, I embarked on a quest to take charge of my health and nutrition. It was a journey marked by learning curves and revelations, one where I discovered the importance of forging a positive relationship with food beyond the simplistic mantra of calorie counting. This book encapsulates that journey, delving into the nuances of nutrition and how it intertwines with our daily lives. It's about more than just the food on our plates; it's about how we engage with food on an emotional, psychological, and social level.

Today, I stand happier in my mindset and enriched by a lifestyle that includes expanded activities, a solid relationship with the right foods, and the freedom to enjoy dinners out and family gatherings without the shadow of guilt. My transformation has ignited a passion within me — a passion for nutrition, well-being, and, most importantly, for helping others who might find themselves in the struggle I once faced.

As we move through the chapters of this book, I'll share insights and strategies that have helped me build a healthier, more joyful relationship with food. It's a narrative that challenges the conventional wisdom of dieting, advocating instead for a balanced approach that doesn't sacrifice the pleasures of eating for health. I hope my story resonates with you, offering guidance and inspiration and perhaps reflecting your journey toward nutritional enlightenment.

I'm thrilled to share what I've learned, buoyed by the hope that my experiences will reach someone who needs this message the most. My journey has evolved into a passion for nutrition and a commitment to helping others navigate their path to wellness. So, as we venture into the heart of this book, remember: this is not just about changing how you eat; it's about transforming how you view and interact with food, paving the way to a healthier, happier you.

Nutrition is not just about counting calories or following the latest diet craze. It's about understanding the building blocks of food — proteins, carbohydrates, and fats — and how they interact with our unique physiological makeup to affect our energy, mood, and overall health. It's about unraveling the mystery of basal metabolic rate (BMR) and why knowing yours is the first step towards tailoring a diet that optimizes your body. It's about recognizing the role of hormones in our dietary choices and the subtle signs of imbalance that we often overlook. It's about acknowledging that supplements and mindset play a crucial role in our nutritional journey.

Who stands to benefit from this book? The answer is simple: anyone and everyone, from teenagers grappling with the pressures of body image to adults navigating the challenges of maintaining a healthy lifestyle amidst a hectic schedule. Whether you're a fitness enthusiast seeking to optimize your energy levels or someone looking to make more informed food choices, this book is designed for you. I aim to equip you with the knowledge and tools to create a balanced, enjoyable eating approach that celebrates life's guilty pleasures without compromising your health.

As we embark on this journey together, I invite you to keep an open mind and a curious heart. The following chapters are structured to build upon each other, starting with the foundational elements of nutrition and advancing toward more complex topics. By the end of this book, you will have a comprehensive understanding of calculating your BMR, differentiating between macronutrients, recognizing the importance of hydration, and much more.

But beyond the science and the strategies, this book is about fostering a relationship with food free from guilt and full of joy. It's about creating a lifestyle that aligns with your needs, preferences, and goals. So, as you turn the page and step into the world of nutritional enlightenment, remember that this journey is not just about the destination. It's about your discoveries, the myths you debunk, and the personal victories you celebrate.

Now, let's turn the page and begin our exploration with a fundamental question that sets the stage for everything that follows: What is a BMR, and how can calculating yours unlock the first door to personalized nutrition?

2

THE BMR AND THE Harris-Benedict Formula

The BMR and the Harris-Benedict Formula

The BMR and the Harris-Benedict Formula: A Deeper Dive

At the heart of personalized nutrition lies an understanding of your Basal Metabolic Rate (BMR), which might seem abstract at first glance but is immensely practical in everyday life. Your BMR is the energy measured in calories your body needs to perform its most basic functions while at rest. These functions are the unsung heroes of your body's daily operations, including breathing, circulating blood, regulating temperature, and cell growth and repair. The silent yet constant energy expenditure keeps you alive without physical activity or digestion.

Why is understanding your BMR so essential? Imagine for a moment that your body is a vehicle. Just as a car requires a baseline amount of fuel to keep its engine running, even when parked, your body needs a certain number of calories to maintain its vital functions at rest. Knowing this baseline helps you understand the minimum amount of fuel (or calories) your body needs before you even factor in additional activities like walking, exercising, or even eating, which all require extra energy.

The significance of BMR extends beyond mere curiosity; it's a critical tool for anyone looking to manage their weight, improve their health, or optimize their physical performance. Calculating your BMR using the Harris-Benedict Formula gives you insight into your body's unique energy demands. This knowledge allows you to tailor your calorie intake more precisely, whether you want to lose weight, gain muscle, or maintain a healthy balance. It serves as your nutritional compass, guiding your diet decisions toward those that support your body's basic needs while accommodating your lifestyle and activity level.

Moreover, understanding your BMR sheds light on the intricate balance of energy metabolism. It helps demystify why some people might lose weight more quickly or struggle to gain weight despite seemingly similar diets and activities. Age, sex, weight, and height all influence your metabolic rate, highlighting the importance of personalized dietary planning over a one-size-fits-all approach.

In essence, your BMR is not just a number; it's a reflection of your body's energy landscape. It underscores the importance of matching your food intake to your body's intrinsic energy requirements, laying the groundwork for informed and effective nutritional strategies. Whether you're embarking on a fitness journey, seeking to enhance your well-being, or simply aiming to understand your body better, calculating your BMR is a vital first step. It empowers you to make choices that align with your body's needs, promoting optimal health and vitality.

Here's a simplified breakdown of how the formula works for both men and women:

- For Men: The formula starts with a base number and then adds calories based on weight, height, and age. It looks like this: 88.362 + (13.397 x your weight in kg) + (4.799 x your height in cm) - (5.677 x your age in years).
- For Women: The formula is slightly different to reflect the general differences in body composition and metabolic rate between sexes: 447.593 + (9.247 x your weight in kg) + (3.098 x your height in cm) - (4.330 x your age in years).

Let's put this into practice with an example:

Imagine a woman who is 30 years old, 5'6" tall (about 167.6 cm), and weighs 140 pounds (about 63.5 kg). Using the formula for women, her BMR calculation would be:

447.593 + (9.247 x 63.5) + (3.098 x 167.6) - (4.330 x 30) = 1,379 calories per day

Without taking any physical activity into account, her body needs approximately 1,379 calories daily to support essential physiological functions.

This was the turning point where the advice I received led me astray. Like many, I was advised by my doctors to simply "eat less and work harder," a piece of guidance that's as common as it is flawed. Contrary to helping, this approach backfired. It triggered my body's defense mechanism, leading it to conserve energy and store fat — the opposite of what I aimed for. Following this, my calorie intake was restricted to less than 800 calories a day, a decision that, in hindsight, did more harm than good. Only through my research and learning did I understand the damage this advice had caused physically and in how my body responded to my efforts. This realization began a journey toward healing and rebuilding the trust between my body and me, highlighting the importance of informed, personalized health strategies.

TDEE-Total Daily Energy Expenditure

we aim to delve deeper into Total Daily Energy Expenditure (TDEE) and explore the significance of identifying your body type to accurately calculate your daily calorie needs, tailoring your nutrition and fitness strategies for maximum effectiveness.

Total Daily Energy Expenditure (TDEE) and the Importance of Body Type

Understanding your Total Daily Energy Expenditure (TDEE) is like unlocking the secret to personalized nutrition and fitness. TDEE represents the total number of calories you burn daily, considering all your activities, from breathing and digesting food (your Basal Metabolic Rate, or BMR) to your job, workouts, and even casual walks. It's a comprehensive snapshot of your calorie expenditure, making it invaluable for anyone looking to manage weight, build muscle, or maintain a healthy lifestyle.

Navigating Nutrition and Fitness Through Body Types

Recognizing your body type isn't just for tailoring your wardrobe; it's crucial for customizing your diet and exercise plans. We can classify body types into three categories: ectomorphs, mesomorphs, and endomorphs. Each has distinct characteristics and metabolic implications.

- **Ectomorphs:** Picture the classic "runner's body" — slim, with a fast metabolism that seems to burn off calories as quickly as they're consumed. Ectomorphs typically have a more petite frame and muscle mass, making it challenging to gain weight or muscle. They might need a higher calorie intake to see muscle growth, emphasizing nutrient-dense foods and strength training to increase their TDEE effectively.
- **Mesomorphs:** These individuals are natural athletes, able to gain muscle and lose fat with relative ease. Mesomorphs have a medium

frame and well-defined muscles, with a metabolism that balances the quick-burning ectomorph and the slower-burning endomorph. For mesomorphs, a balanced diet rich in proteins, carbohydrates, and fats, combined with a mix of strength and cardiovascular training, can optimize their TDEE for muscle building or weight management.

- **Endomorphs**: Endomorphs have a larger bone structure and a higher total body and fat mass. Their metabolism is slower, making weight gain easy but weight loss challenging. To effectively manage their TDEE, endomorphs may focus on a lower calorie intake, higher protein, and fiber to enhance satiety and incorporate regular cardio and strength training to boost their metabolic rate.

Understanding your body type allows for a nuanced approach to calculating your TDEE. It's not just about the calories burned during a gym session; it's about how your body conserves or expends energy throughout the day, influenced by your genetic predisposition. By aligning your nutrition and exercise regimen with your body type, you can create a tailored strategy that supports your health goals, whether losing fat, building muscle, or enhancing overall wellness.

In summary, your TDEE and body type are instrumental in crafting a personalized health and fitness plan. By acknowledging the unique aspects of your body type, you can adjust your calorie intake and exercise strategies to suit your metabolic needs, propelling you toward your goals with greater precision and success.

SUGGESTED CALORIE INTAKE-Body Type, Calorie Intake, and Macronutrient Breakdown

We dive into the specific calorie and macronutrient recommendations tailored to each body type, providing a framework for crafting a diet that aligns with your unique metabolic needs and fitness goals.

The foundation of any effective nutrition plan lies in understanding how many calories to consume and the quality and distribution of those calories across macronutrients: proteins, carbohydrates, and fats. Each body type has distinct requirements that can guide these decisions.

Ectomorph: The High-Energy Dynamo

Ectomorphs are lean, often taller individuals who struggle to gain weight or muscle mass due to their fast metabolism. They thrive on a high-carbohydrate diet that supports their energy needs.

- Macronutrient Prescription:
- Carbohydrates: 55-60% of total calorie intake
- Protein: 25-30%
- Fats: 15-20%

Goal: To fuel workouts and muscle recovery while accommodating a rapid metabolism.

Mesomorph: The Versatile Athlete

Mesomorphs have a naturally athletic build, finding it more accessible to gain muscle and control body fat. They benefit from a balanced distribution of macronutrients supporting muscle gain and fat loss.

- Macronutrient Prescription:
- Carbohydrates: 40-50% of total calorie intake
- Protein: 30%
- Fats: 20-30%

Goal: To maintain muscle mass and energy levels while staying lean.

Endomorph: The Strength Builder

Endomorphs tend to have a larger frame and may gain weight easily. They excel on a diet lower in carbohydrates but higher in protein and fats, which can help manage body fat levels while supporting muscle growth.

- Macronutrient Prescription:
- Carbohydrates: 25-30% of total calorie intake
- Protein: 35-40%
- Fats: 30-35%

Goal: To enhance satiety, support metabolism, and encourage fat loss while building muscle.

Implementing Your Macro Prescription

- Calculate Your Caloric Needs: First, determine your Total Daily Energy Expenditure (TDEE) to understand how many calories you need to maintain weight. Adjust this number based on your goals (e.g., add calories for muscle gain, subtract for fat loss).
- Apply Your Macro Prescription: Based on your body type and caloric needs, divide your total calorie intake according to the percentages for your macronutrient prescription.
- Adjust and Monitor: Your body's response is your ultimate guide. Monitor your progress and adjust your macronutrient ratios as needed, depending on how your body responds to the diet.

Example of a Mesomorph Aiming for Muscle Gain:

If the TDEE is 2,500 calories and the goal is muscle gain, adding an extra 500 calories would result in a total of 3,000 calories per day.

- Carbohydrates: 40% of 3,000 calories = 1,200 calories / 4 kcal per gram = 300 grams

- Protein: 30% of 3,000 calories = 900 calories / 4 kcal per gram = 225 grams
- Fats: 30% of 3,000 calories = 900 calories / 9 kcal per gram = 100 grams

Calculating Your Needs

First, determine your TDEE based on your body type and activity level to calculate your needs. Then, adjust your calorie intake according to your goals (gain muscle, lose fat, maintain weight) and distribute these calories across macronutrients.

For example, an ectomorph aiming to gain muscle might calculate their TDEE as 2,500 calories and choose to consume 3,000 calories daily for a surplus. If they follow a macro split of 55% carbs, 25% protein, and 20% fats, their daily targets would be approximately 412 grams of carbs, 188 grams of protein, and 67 grams of fats.

Remember, these recommendations are starting points. Monitoring your body's response and adjusting your intake and macronutrient distribution as needed is important. Keeping a food and activity journal can be incredibly helpful in tracking progress and making informed adjustments to your plan.

Here's a streamlined approach to understanding how to tailor your macronutrient intake according to your body type, ensuring you feed your muscles and achieve your fitness goals efficiently. Each body type—ectomorph, mesomorph, and endomorph—has unique nutritional needs that, when met with precision, can significantly enhance muscle growth, fat loss, and overall health.

This macro prescription ensures the mesomorph has enough energy for workouts, protein for muscle repair and growth, and fats for hormonal health and nutrient absorption. Tailoring your diet this way can be a game-changer in achieving your fitness and body composition goals. Remember, consistency, patience, and regular adjustments based on your progress are crucial to success.

Conclusion: Harnessing the Power of BMR, TDEE, and Body Types for Tailored Nutrition

Embarking on a journey to optimize your health and fitness through nutrition is both a science and an art. By understanding the foundational concepts of Basal Metabolic Rate (BMR) and Total Daily Energy Expenditure (TDEE) and recognizing the influence of body types on metabolic needs, you've taken the first critical steps toward personalizing your nutritional strategy. These key insights allow you to confidently navigate the complex landscape of dietary planning, ensuring that your food intake is sufficient and ideally attuned to your body's unique requirements.

Calculating your BMR gives you a glimpse into the inner workings of your body at rest, offering a baseline for the calories needed to support vital functions. Extending this understanding to include TDEE incorporates the dynamic aspects of your lifestyle and physical activity, providing a comprehensive view of your total caloric needs. Furthermore, acknowledging the significance of body types—whether you're an ectomorph, mesomorph, or endomorph—adds another layer of customization, enabling you to fine-tune your calorie and macronutrient intake to support your specific goals, whether it's weight loss, muscle gain, or maintaining your current physique.

The suggested caloric and macronutrient breakdowns for each body type serve as a guide to help you craft a diet that complements your metabolic profile and fitness ambitions. However, remember that these recommendations are starting points. The true essence of a successful nutrition plan lies in its adaptability—listening to your body, observing how it responds to different adjustments, and being willing to refine your approach as you progress. Nutrition is deeply personal, and what works for one individual may not work for another, highlighting the importance of patience, persistence, and a willingness to experiment.

In conclusion, you can embark on a personalized nutrition journey armed with your BMR, TDEE, and body type knowledge. This journey is not just about the numbers but about developing a deeper connection with your body, understanding its signals, and respecting its needs. By aligning your dietary intake with your body's intrinsic energy requirements and goals, you can create a harmonious balance that supports optimal health, vitality, and well-being. Remember, the path to achieving your fitness and health objectives is not linear; it's a continuous learning, adjusting, and growing process. Embrace this journey with an open heart and mind, and let the principles of BMR, TDEE, and body type guide you toward a healthier, more fulfilled life.

3

UNDERSTANDING OUR ENERGY SYSTEM: The Thermic Effect of Feeding (TEF) and Calorie Expenditure

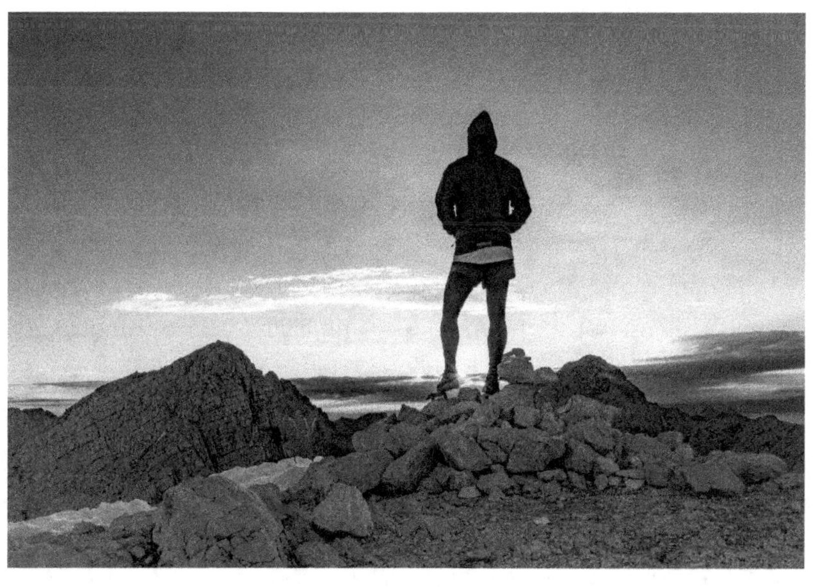

The Thermic Effect of Feeding (TEF) is a critical component of our body's total daily energy expenditure (TDEE), representing the energy expended to process food. It accounts for about 10% of TDEE, varying with the macronutrient composition of our meals. Here's why it matters:

- Protein's High TEF: Protein supports muscle repair and growth and has a high thermic effect, with 20-30% of protein calories burned during digestion. This makes protein-rich diets beneficial for weight management, as they can boost metabolic rate and increase feelings of fullness, potentially leading to a natural reduction in calorie intake.
- Carbohydrates and Fats: Carbohydrates have a moderate thermic effect (5-10%), while fats have the lowest (0-3%). This doesn't mean fats and carbs are "bad," but balancing your intake with a higher proportion of protein can enhance TDEE through TEF.
- Strategic Meal Planning: Leveraging TEF can inform more thoughtful meal planning. For instance, a protein source in each meal can elevate your metabolic rate more than a meal heavy in carbs or fats. This doesn't imply extreme dietary restrictions but suggests a balanced approach for optimal metabolic efficiency.
- Implications for Weight Management: Understanding TEF can be a game-changer in weight management strategies. It emphasizes the importance of meal composition over just calorie counting. By focusing on nutrient-dense foods and balancing macronutrients, you can support your body's energy expenditure and weight management goals more effectively.

Incorporating this knowledge into your dietary strategy can make a noticeable difference in how your body processes food and manages weight. It underscores the significance of how much we eat and what we eat, highlighting the synergy between diet composition and metabolic health.

Understanding Non-exercise Activity Thermogenesis (NEAT)

Non-exercise Activity Thermogenesis, or NEAT, is the energy we expend for everything that's not sleeping, eating, or formal exercise. This includes walking to the mailbox, vacuuming the living room, or tapping your foot while seated. The fascinating part about NEAT is its significant variance among individuals, leading to a daily caloric difference of up to 2,000 calories between two people with similar sedentary jobs.

Consider Sarah, a graphic designer who works from home. She consciously integrates more activity into her day: opting for a standing desk, taking short walks every hour, and always using the stairs in her two-story house. These seemingly minor changes have increased her daily calorie burn and contributed to her overall weight management strategy without ever stepping into a gym.

Sarah's example underscores the potential of NEAT in enhancing metabolic health and aiding weight control. Simple lifestyle adjustments to stay more active throughout the day can significantly boost your NEAT, offering an accessible way to improve your health and well-being

Exercise Activity Thermogenesis (EAT) Detailed

Exercise Activity Thermogenesis (EAT) encompasses the energy expended during all planned and structured physical activities, ranging from a morning run to an intense session at the gym. Unlike the passive calories burned through daily movements, or NEAT, EAT results from conscious decisions to engage in activities that elevate the heart rate, challenge the muscles, and boost overall energy expenditure.

The impact of EAT on an individual's daily calorie burn is significant and highly variable, deeply influenced by the type, intensity, and duration of the exercises performed. For instance, a 30-minute high-intensity interval training (HIIT) session can burn substantially different calories compared to a 30-minute yoga practice due to differences in intensity and muscle engagement.

Take, for example, Alex and Jordan:

- Alex enjoys brisk walking for an hour each day, which might burn approximately 300 calories, contributing to his EAT and overall calorie deficit for weight management.
- Jordan, on the other hand, prefers weightlifting and spends about an hour in the gym on a routine that can torch upwards of 500 calories, significantly enhancing his EAT and facilitating muscle growth and fat loss.

Regularly incorporating exercise into one's routine increases EAT and yields numerous health benefits, including improved heart health, stronger muscles, better mood, and enhanced metabolic efficiency. For individuals focused on weight management or muscle gain, understanding and optimizing EAT through tailored exercise plans becomes crucial to their overall strategy, allowing for a more directed and effective approach to achieving their fitness goals.

Aerobic Training

Aerobic training is a cornerstone of fitness, focusing on continuous, rhythmic activities that elevate your heart rate and breathing over time. Its primary aim is to boost the cardiovascular system's efficiency, enhancing oxygen uptake and delivery throughout the body. Key benefits of aerobic exercise include:

- Enhanced cardiovascular health
- Increased lung capacity
- Improved endurance and stamina
- Significant calorie burn
- Lowered risk of chronic diseases
- Mental health benefits

Example:

- Maria's Routine: Maria, a 35-year-old to improve her cardiovascular health and lose weight, incorporates aerobic training into her weekly routine. She opts for:
- Brisk Walking: 30 minutes during her lunch break on weekdays.
- Cycling: A 45-minute session on weekends at a moderate pace.

This structured approach allows Maria to increase her daily calorie expenditure significantly, improve her heart health, and build endurance, demonstrating the versatility and effectiveness of aerobic training in achieving fitness goals.

Anaerobic Training

Anaerobic training is characterized by high-intensity activities performed in short bursts, where the body's demand for oxygen surpasses the oxygen supply available. It primarily uses the body's internal energy stores as fuel, making it excellent for building muscle strength and improving overall athletic performance. Common anaerobic exercises include sprinting, lifting weights, and high-intensity interval training

(HIIT).

Example:

- Lena's Strength Plan: To enhance her physical strength and muscle tone, Lena engages in anaerobic training sessions that focus on:
- Heavy Weight Lifting: Targeting different muscle groups with heavy weights for low repetitions, three times a week.
- HIIT Workouts: Incorporating 20-minute high-intensity interval training sessions twice weekly, alternating between full effort and rest periods.

Lena's structured anaerobic workouts boost her muscular endurance and power and significantly contribute to her metabolic rate, aiding in more effective fat-burning and muscle definition.

The key differences between aerobic and anaerobic training are their intensity, duration, energy sources, and overall health benefits. Here's a breakdown to clarify these distinctions:

Aerobic Training

- Intensity & Duration: Aerobic exercises are typically moderate in intensity and longer in duration. They are designed to increase the heart rate and breathing for extended periods.
- Energy Source: Uses oxygen to fuel the body for the activity. The body burns fats and carbohydrates with oxygen to produce energy.
- Benefits: Improves cardiovascular health, increases stamina and endurance, promotes fat burning, and improves mental health due to the release of endorphins.
- Examples: Running, cycling, swimming, and brisk walking.

Anaerobic Training

- Intensity & Duration: Anaerobic exercises are high in intensity but short in duration. They involve quick bursts of energy and are performed with maximum effort for a brief period.
- Energy Source: Relies on the body's internal energy stores (like ATP and glycogen) instead of oxygen for short, intense bursts of activity. This leads to the production of lactate.
- Benefits: Increases muscle strength, power, and size; enhances the body's resting metabolic rate; improves speed and power; and boosts muscle endurance.
- Examples: Sprinting, heavy weight lifting, and high-intensity interval training (HIIT).

In summary, while aerobic training focuses on improving endurance and cardiovascular health through prolonged activities fueled by oxygen, anaerobic training targets muscle strength, size, and power through short, high-intensity bursts that rely on the body's internal energy reserves. Both forms of exercise offer unique benefits and can be combined in a well-rounded fitness program to achieve comprehensive health and fitness goals.

Integrating both aerobic and anaerobic training into your daily routine can maximize your health benefits, improve physical fitness, and ensure a balanced approach to your workouts. Here's how you can effectively incorporate these exercises into your daily life:

Establishing a Routine

- Set Clear Goals: Determine what you aim to achieve with your fitness routine, be it weight loss, muscle gain, improved endurance, or overall health. Your goals will dictate the balance of aerobic and anaerobic exercises in your regimen.

- Create a Schedule: Plan your week. Allocate specific days for aerobic training and others for anaerobic training. For example, you might do aerobic exercises like running or cycling on Mondays, Wednesdays, and Fridays and reserve Tuesdays and Thursdays for anaerobic workouts such as weight lifting or HIIT.

Daily Integration Tips

- Aerobic Training:
- Morning Routine: Start your day with a brisk walk or a light jog. Morning aerobic activity can boost your metabolism and energy levels throughout the day.
- Commute Considerations: If possible, cycle or walk to work. It's an excellent way to incorporate aerobic exercise into your daily routine without needing extra time at the gym.
- Anaerobic Training:
- Lunch Break Workouts: Utilize a part of your lunch break for a quick session of bodyweight exercises or sprints near your workplace.
- Evening Sessions: Engage in strength training or HIIT in the evening. This can also help you unwind and relieve the stress of the day.

Combining Both for Optimal Results

- Alternate Days: To prevent overtraining and ensure adequate recovery, alternate between aerobic and anaerobic workouts throughout the week.
- Incorporate Active Recovery: On days following intense anaerobic sessions, consider light aerobic activity, such as a gentle bike ride or a swim, to help your muscles recover while remaining active.

- Listen to Your Body: Adjust the intensity and frequency of your workouts based on your body's feelings. Rest is just as important as the workouts themselves.

Lifestyle Considerations

- Stay Active Outside the Gym: Look for opportunities to be active in everyday life—take the stairs instead of the elevator, play with your kids at the park, or engage in a hobby that keeps you moving.
- Nutrition and Hydration: Support your exercise routine with a balanced diet and plenty of water. Nutrition plays a crucial role in energy levels and recovery.

By thoughtfully integrating aerobic and anaerobic exercises into your daily life, you can enjoy the full spectrum of health benefits these activities offer. Remember, consistency is key, and finding activities you enjoy will help you maintain a balanced and active lifestyle in the long term.

This chapter has provided a detailed look at how our bodies expend energy through the Thermic Effect of Feeding (TEF), Non-exercise Activity Thermogenesis (NEAT), and Exercise Activity Thermogenesis (EAT). Understanding these concepts is crucial for anyone looking to manage weight, improve metabolic health, or enhance physical fitness. Here are the practical steps and strategies you can take based on what we've covered:

- Leverage TEF: Optimize your diet for the thermic effect by increasing your intake of proteins, which have a higher thermic effect than fats and carbohydrates. This can aid in weight management and metabolic rate improvement.

- Increase NEAT: Incorporate more physical activity into your daily routine outside of structured exercise. Simple changes like taking the stairs, walking for short errands, or standing while working can significantly increase your daily calorie expenditure.
- Balance EAT: Integrate a mix of aerobic and anaerobic exercises into your weekly fitness routine. Aerobic exercises improve cardiovascular health and endurance, while anaerobic exercises are key for building strength and muscle mass.

Here's how you can apply these insights:

- For TEF: Include a protein source in every meal. This could be lean meats, legumes, or dairy products.
- For NEAT: Set reminders to stand up or move around every hour if you have a sedentary job. Consider a walking meeting instead of a sit-down one.
- For EAT: Plan your exercise week with three days of weight training (anaerobic) and two days of cardio (aerobic). Adjust based on your goals and recovery.

Remember, the goal is to make informed choices that suit your lifestyle and fitness goals. The understanding of TEF, NEAT, and EAT provides a foundation for these decisions, empowering you to manage your energy expenditure effectively. As you apply these strategies, monitor your progress and be prepared to adjust your approach as needed. This chapter isn't just theory—it's a practical guide to improving your health and fitness.

4

MACRONUTRIENT , VITAMINS AND PROTEIN

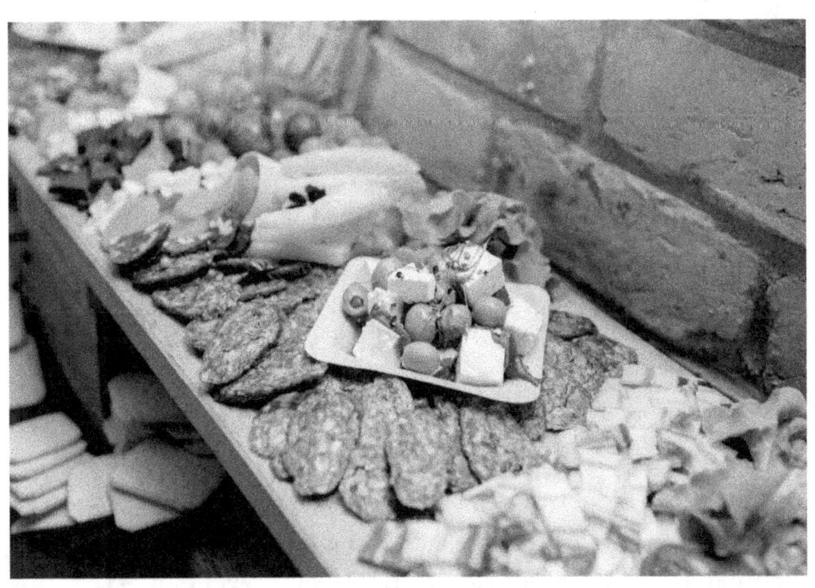

A Practical Guide to Protein in Your Diet

Protein is a fundamental macronutrient for everyone, not just athletes or fitness enthusiasts. It's crucial for repairing tissues, making hormones and enzymes, and supporting immune function. Here's a straightforward look at why protein is vital and how you can effectively incorporate it into your diet.

The Significance of Protein

- Essential for Muscle Repair: Important for anyone engaging in physical activity, protein helps repair and build muscle tissue.
- Supports Bodily Functions: Proteins are necessary for creating hormones and enzymes that regulate body processes.
- Boosts Immune Health: Proteins form antibodies that help fight off infections.
- Facilitates Oxygen Transport: The protein hemoglobin carries oxygen throughout the body, supporting cellular function.

Vitamins That Enhance Protein Use

Specific vitamins are essential for protein utilization:

- Vitamin B6: Necessary for metabolizing protein and producing neurotransmitters. It is found in poultry, fish, and potatoes.
- Vitamin B12: Critical for protein synthesis and red blood cell formation. Available in meat, fish, and fortified cereals.
- Vitamin D Helps muscle function and works with calcium to strengthen bones. Get it from sunlight exposure, fatty fish, or fortified dairy.

How to Include Protein in Your Diet

- Understand Protein Sources: Know that animal proteins (meat, fish, dairy) contain all essential amino acids, while plant-based sources (legumes, grains) might need to be combined to offer a complete protein profile.
- Eggs Are Efficient: Eggs provide a complete set of essential amino acids, making them an excellent protein source.
- Explore Plant Proteins: Foods like quinoa, hemp seeds, and peas are great plant-based protein options.

To ensure you're getting enough protein:

- Include a protein source in every meal, aiming for variety to cover all essential amino acids.
- Consider your lifestyle and activity level when determining how much protein you need. Active individuals may require more protein for muscle repair and recovery.
- Pair plant-based proteins to form complete proteins if you follow a vegetarian or vegan diet, ensuring you get all essential amino acids.

Incorporating various protein sources and vitamin-rich foods that aid in protein metabolism can optimize your health and support your body's needs. Keep your diet diverse to maximize proteins' benefits, and adjust your intake based on your health goals and physical activity levels.

Here are some fun facts about protein and its role in our diet and body:

- 1. Hair and Nails are Mostly Protein: Keratin, a type of protein, is a significant component of your hair and nails. Adequate protein intake can help keep them strong and healthy.

- 2. Protein is Everywhere in Your Body: Aside from water, protein is the most abundant substance in your body, present in everything from muscles and organs to enzymes and hormones.
- 3. The Word "Protein" Comes from the Greek Word "Protos": Meaning "first," protein is named for its top-tier importance in the body's structure and function.
- 4. There Are 20 Different Amino Acids: Your body uses these amino acids to build and repair tissues. While the body produces 11, 9 are essential and must come from your diet.
- 5. Not All Proteins Are Equal: The quality of a protein is determined by its amino acid composition. Animal proteins are considered "complete" because they contain all essential amino acids, while most plant proteins are "incomplete," lacking one or more.
- 6. The First Protein Structure was Discovered in 1958: John Kendrew mapped the structure of myoglobin, a protein that stores oxygen in muscle cells, marking a significant milestone in biochemistry.
- 7. Cheese is Protein-Rich: Hard cheeses like Parmesan are among the highest protein-containing foods, with about 35.1 grams of protein per 100 grams.
- 8. Ancient Proteins Tell Us About Prehistoric Life: Scientists study ancient proteins found in fossils to understand more about extinct animals and humans, including their diets and environments.
- 9. Protein Can Help You Feel Full: Thanks to its slow digestion, protein can help you feel fuller longer, making it an essential macronutrient for managing hunger and weight.
- 10. Quinoa is a Complete Protein: Among plant-based foods, quinoa stands out because it contains all nine essential amino acids, making it an excellent protein source for vegetarians and vegans.

These fun facts underscore the crucial role of protein in not just nutrition but in the fundamental aspects of biology and history. Whether you're adjusting your diet for health, fitness, or curiosity, protein is a fascinating and essential component of life.

The protein you need daily depends on several key factors, like weight, activity level, and health goals. Generally, the dietary recommendation is to consume 0.8 grams of protein per kilogram of body weight if you're sedentary. However, if you're active or aim to build muscle, your protein needs increase, ranging from 1.2 to 2.0 grams per kilogram.

Examples of protein Sources:

Animal-Based Protein Sources:

- Chicken breast
- Turkey
- Eggs
- Greek yogurt
- Milk
- Cheese
- Beef
- Pork
- Fish, such as salmon, tuna, and trout
- Shrimp

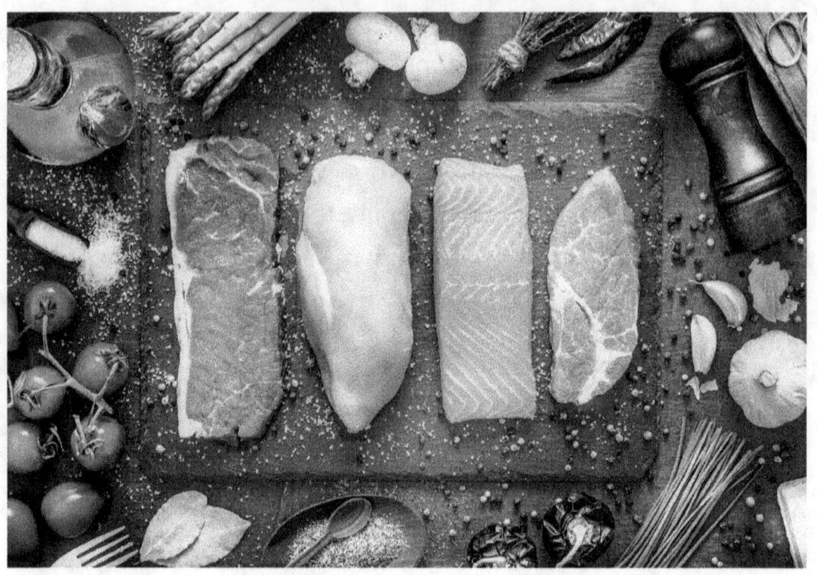

Plant-Based Protein Sources:

- Lentils
- Chickpeas
- Black beans
- Quinoa
- Tofu
- Tempeh
- Edamame
- Hemp seeds
- Chia seeds
- Nut butters, such as almond or peanut butter

Including various protein sources in your diet can help you get a wide range of essential amino acids and other nutrients.

Practical Protein Intake Examples

- For a Sedentary Individual:
- Case: Sarah, a 68 kg (150 lbs) woman who exercises lightly, needs about 54 grams of protein daily.
- Daily Protein Strategy:
- Breakfast: A smoothie with protein powder (20g protein)
- Lunch: A turkey sandwich (20g protein)
- Dinner: Lentil soup (14g protein)
- Total: 54 grams of protein, aligning perfectly with her daily requirement.
- For an Active Person:
- Case: Mike, an 80 kg (176 lbs) man engaging in heavy lifting and cardio, targets around 1.5g/kg, equating to 120 grams of protein daily.
- Daily Protein Strategy:
- Breakfast: Oatmeal with almond butter and a side of eggs (30g protein)
- Lunch: Grilled chicken salad (40g protein)
- Snack: Greek yogurt (20g protein)
- Dinner: Beef stir-fry with veggies (30g protein)
- Total: 120 grams of protein, supporting his active lifestyle and muscle-building goals.

These scenarios show how to meet protein needs based on individual lifestyles and goals.

For sedentary individuals, focusing on balanced meals with moderate protein sources is key. **Active individuals** or those building muscle should prioritize higher protein intakes across meals and snacks, incorporating a mix of animal and plant-based proteins to ensure all essential amino acids are consumed. Adjusting portion sizes and protein sources can help meet the precise protein requirements without overcomplicating meal planning.

Protein deficiency, though rare in developed countries, can occur under certain circumstances, such as with restrictive diets, in older adults, or those with specific health conditions. Recognizing the signs and symptoms of protein deficiency is crucial for addressing this issue before it leads to more serious health problems.

PROTEIN DEFICIENCY

Signs and Symptoms of Protein Deficiency:

- Muscle Loss and Weakness: Protein is essential for building and repairing muscle tissue. A deficiency can lead to muscle atrophy and weakness.
- Skin, Hair, and Nail Problems: You might notice brittle nails, hair thinning or loss, and skin issues due to the lack of protein, which is vital for their health and renewal.
- Increased Susceptibility to Infections: Proteins play a crucial role in the immune system. A deficiency can weaken your immune response, making you more susceptible to infections.
- Edema: Lack of protein can cause fluid imbalance, leading to swelling, especially in the feet and ankles.
- Feeling Tired and Weak: Without enough protein, your body lacks the resources to produce energy efficiently, leading to persistent fatigue.
- Hunger and Appetite Changes: Protein helps regulate hunger by promoting feelings of fullness. A deficiency might lead to increased

hunger and overeating.

- Slow Healing of Wounds: Protein is crucial for the healing process, and a deficiency can slow down the repair of wounds and injuries.
- Bone Fractures: Protein supports bone health, and a deficiency can lead to weaker bones and an increased risk of fractures.

Long-term Consequences of Protein Deficiency:

If not addressed, protein deficiency can lead to more severe health issues, including:

- Severe Malnutrition: Known as kwashiorkor in children, which can be fatal if untreated.
- Growth Failure: A lack of protein can severely impact growth and development in children.
- Immune System Dysfunction: Leading to an increased risk of severe infections and illnesses.
- Cardiovascular Problems: Protein is vital for a healthy heart and circulatory system. A deficiency can lead to cardiovascular issues.
- Respiratory Issues: Weak respiratory muscles due to protein deficiency can affect lung function and breathing.

Addressing protein deficiency involves increasing protein intake through diet. This can be achieved by incorporating protein-rich foods such as meats, dairy products, legumes, and grains. In some cases, supplements might be recommended. However, consulting with a healthcare provider or nutritionist is crucial to identify the deficiency's underlying cause and develop an appropriate treatment plan.

CONCLUSION

Concluding our discussion on protein, it's evident that this macronutrient is fundamental to maintaining and improving overall health. Protein deficiency, though rare in well-nourished societies, poses serious health risks ranging from muscle loss to weakened immunity when it does occur. Identifying signs of deficiency early and addressing them through dietary adjustments is key to preventing long-term health issues.

The takeaway is clear: ensuring adequate protein intake is essential for everyone, regardless of lifestyle or dietary preferences. Whether through animal or plant sources, a varied and balanced diet can meet your protein needs, supporting everything from muscle repair to immune function.

In summary, the importance of protein in the diet cannot be overstated. Being mindful of your protein intake and making necessary adjustments based on your health status, activity level, and dietary restrictions will support your overall well-being. Keep protein's role in mind as you plan your meals and make dietary choices, aiming for a balanced intake to maintain optimal health.

5

MACRONUTRIENTS -FATS

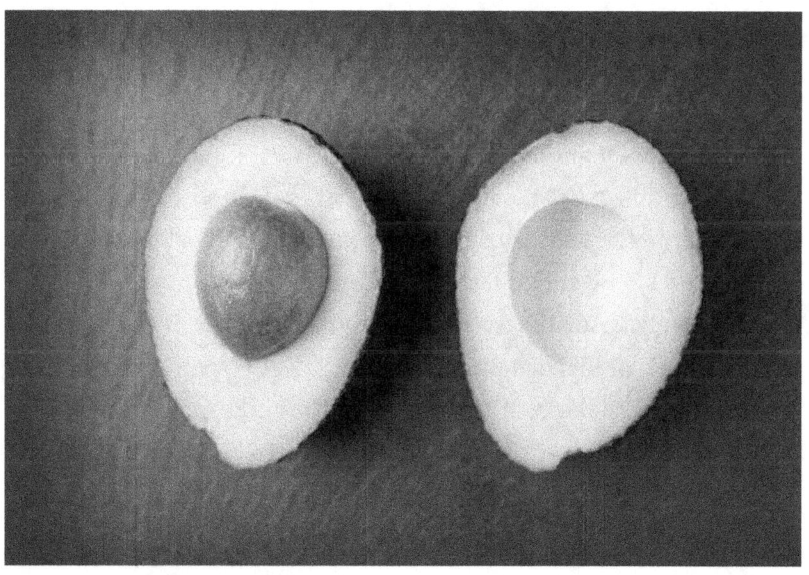

Fats: The Essential Macronutrient:

Fats are crucial dietary components that play multifaceted roles in maintaining and enhancing bodily functions. Often misunderstood and wrongly vilified, fats are, in fact, vital for a plethora of bodily processes, from serving as a significant energy reservoir to ensuring the smooth operation of cellular mechanisms. Here's an in-depth look at the indispensable benefits of fats and where to find them:

- -Major Energy Source: Fats provide a substantial energy yield of 9 calories per gram, making them the most energy-dense macronutrient. This energy is vital during prolonged, low to moderate-intensity physical activities and supports the body's metabolic functions during rest.
- Cellular Integrity and Function: Every cell in our body is encased in a lipid membrane. These lipids maintain the fluidity and flexibility of cell membranes, allowing for the proper flow of nutrients into cells and waste products.
- -Absorption of Fat-Soluble Vitamins: Fats aid in absorbing vitamins A, D, E, and K, which are crucial for vision, bone health, antioxidant functions, and blood clotting, respectively. Our bodies cannot effectively absorb these nutrients without sufficient dietary fats, regardless of their intake levels.
- -Hormonal Balance: Fats contribute to synthesizing various hormones, including sex hormones like estrogen and testosterone, and hormones involved in metabolism regulation. These hormonal activities influence growth, reproductive health, and metabolic rates.

Sources and Types of Beneficial Fats:

- Monounsaturated Fats: Found in olive oil, avocados, and certain nuts (like almonds and peanuts), these fats can improve heart health by reducing harmful cholesterol levels and increasing good cholesterol.
- Polyunsaturated Fats: These include omega-3 and omega-6 fatty acids found in fatty fish (salmon, mackerel, sardines), flaxseeds, and walnuts. Omega-3s are mainly known for their anti-inflammatory properties and their role in heart health and brain function.
- Saturated Fats: While often depicted negatively, saturated fats, found in dairy products, red meat, and coconut oil, play roles in brain health and the integrity of cell membranes. However, moderation is key, as excessive intake can contribute to heart disease.

Understanding the critical roles of fats in the body underscores the importance of including healthy fats in your diet. By choosing sources rich in monounsaturated and polyunsaturated fats and consuming saturated fats in moderation, you can support your body's energy needs, cellular health, nutrient absorption, and hormonal balance, contributing to overall well-being and disease prevention.

Healthy Fats vs. Unhealthy Fats

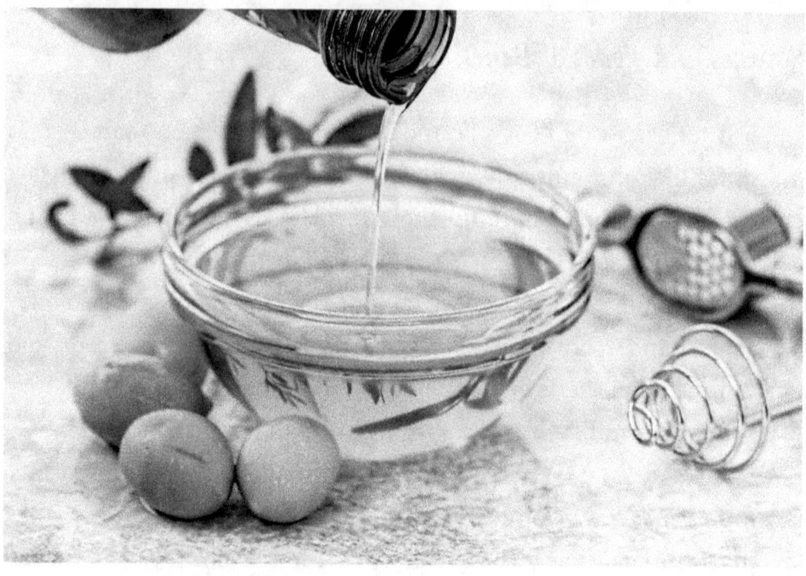

Incorporating suitable types of fats into your diet is crucial for optimal health. Here's a quick guide on healthy and unhealthy fat sources, followed by an explanation of brown fat.

Healthy Fats:

- **Monounsaturated Fats:**
- Sources: Olive oil, avocados, almonds, pecans, and sesame seeds.
- Benefits: Improve heart health by reducing bad LDL cholesterol levels and increasing good HDL cholesterol.
- **Polyunsaturated Fats** (including Omega-3 and Omega-6 fatty acids):
- Sources: Fatty fish (salmon, mackerel, sardines), flaxseeds, walnuts, and sunflower seeds.
- Benefits: Essential for brain function and cell growth. Omega-3s

help reduce inflammation and are linked to a lower risk of heart disease.

Unhealthy Fats:

- **Saturated Fats:**
- Sources: Red meat, butter, cheese, and coconut oil.
- Note: While necessary in small amounts, excessive intake can raise total and LDL cholesterol levels, increasing the risk of heart disease. Moderation is key.
- **Trans Fats:**
- Sources: Processed foods, baked goods, and some fried foods.
- Health Risks: Increase LDL cholesterol, reduce HDL cholesterol, and are linked to a higher risk of heart disease and stroke

Brown Fat:

- What is Brown Fat?:
- Brown adipose tissue, or brown fat, is a type of fat that generates heat to help maintain body temperature in cold conditions. It's called "brown" because of its dark color due to the high number of mitochondria containing iron.
- Function and Health Benefits:
- Unlike white fat, which stores energy, brown fat burns calories to produce heat, making it a potential ally in weight management and obesity prevention.
- Research suggests that activating brown fat can improve glucose metabolism and insulin sensitivity, further protecting against diabetes and obesity.
- How to Activate Brown Fat:
- Exposure to cold temperatures can stimulate brown fat activity.

Short periods of cold exposure, such as cold showers or spending time in cooler environments, may help activate brown fat.
- Exercise may also stimulate hormone production that activates brown fat.

Understanding the differences between healthy and unhealthy fats can guide you in making informed dietary choices that support heart health, reduce inflammation, and contribute to overall well-being. Meanwhile, the unique properties of brown fat offer exciting possibilities for metabolic health and weight management, highlighting the complex and beneficial roles that different types of fat play in our bodies.

FAT INTAKE RECOMMENDATIONS

The dietary recommendation for fat intake varies depending on overall caloric needs but generally falls between 20% to 35% of total daily calories. This means, that for an average adult consuming a 2,000-calorie diet, fat intake should range from 44 to 77 **grams per** day. Here's how you can meet these recommendations, along with examples and fun facts:

Recommendations for Fat Intake:

- Choose Healthy Fats: Prioritize monounsaturated and polyunsaturated fats, including omega-3 fatty acids, for their heart-health benefits.
- Examples: Add a handful of almonds (about 14 grams of fat) or a tablespoon of olive oil (about 14 grams of fat) to your meals.
- Limit Saturated Fats: Keep saturated fat intake to less than 10% of total daily calories to support heart health.
- Examples: Opt for lean cuts of meat and choose dairy products that

are low in fat.

- Avoid Trans Fats: Aim to eliminate trans fats from your diet, as they are linked to an increased risk of heart disease.
- Examples: Steer clear of processed foods and snacks that list "partially hydrogenated oils" in their ingredients.

Fun Facts:

- *Did You Know?: The human brain is nearly 60% fat, making dietary fats crucial for brain health and cognitive function.*
- *A Historical Snack: The avocado, rich in monounsaturated fats, was so valued by the Aztecs that they named it āhuacatl, which also meant "testicle" due to its shape.*
- *Omega-3 Power: Omega-3 fatty acids, found in fatty fish like salmon, can improve heart health and enhance mood and cognitive performance.*

Practical Tips:

- Morning Boost: Start your day with a smoothie with chia seeds or flaxseeds rich in omega-3s.
- Snack Smart: For a healthy snack, try a small portion of nuts like walnuts or almonds, or snack on olives, which are high in monounsaturated fats.
- Cooking Choices: Use olive oil for cooking and salad dressings; it's a heart-healthy fat that can withstand moderate cooking temperatures.

By incorporating a variety of healthy fats into your diet and being mindful of the balance between different types of fats, you can support your overall health while enjoying the rich flavors they add to food. Fats are essential to a balanced diet, contributing to satiety, nutrient absorption, and cellular health.

CONCLUSION

Concluding this chapter on fats, it's clear that fats play an indispensable role in our diet, essential for providing energy, supporting cell health, aiding in the absorption of vitamins, and contributing to hormone synthesis. The goal is to ensure that 20% to 35% of your daily caloric intake comes from fats, prioritizing healthy sources like monounsaturated and polyunsaturated fats, particularly omega-3 fatty acids, while minimizing saturated fats and eliminating trans fats. Opt for foods rich in healthy fats such as avocados, nuts, and olive oil to enjoy their myriad health benefits, from cardiovascular health to improved cognitive function. Balancing your fat intake is key to a nutritious diet and long-term well-being.

6

MACRONUTRIENT CARBOHYDRATES

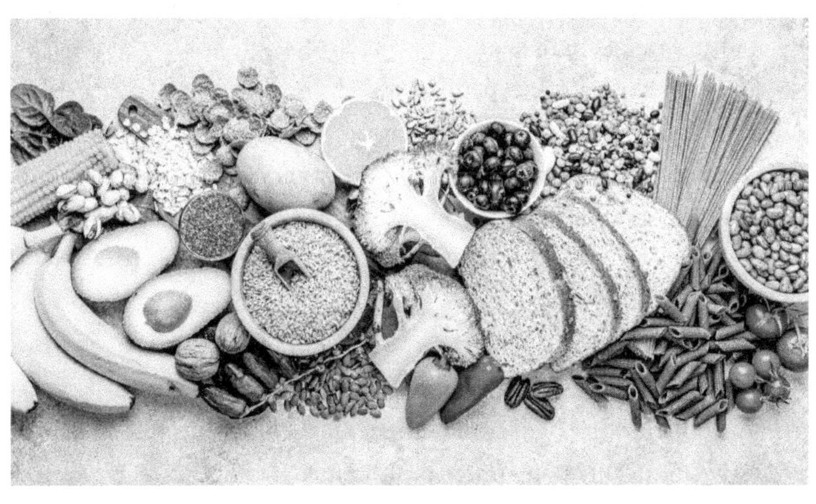

Carbohydrates: Simple, Complex, and the Role of Fiber

Carbohydrates, categorized into simple and complex forms,

are a primary energy source for the body. However, carbohydrates are not considered an essential macronutrient, unlike proteins and fats. This classification is based on the body's ability to generate glucose, a key energy source, through other means when carbohydrate intake is low.

- Simple Carbohydrates: These are quickly digested and absorbed, providing immediate energy. Simple sugars are found in fruits, dairy, and refined sugars. While they offer a quick energy boost, their consumption can lead to rapid spikes in blood sugar levels.
- Complex Carbohydrates: Comprising longer chains of sugar molecules, complex carbohydrates are digested more slowly, gradually releasing energy. They are found in whole grains, legumes, and starchy vegetables, helping to maintain stable blood sugar levels and sustained energy.
- Fiber: Technically a type of complex carbohydrate, fiber is indigestible by the human body. It plays a crucial role in digestive health, helps regulate blood sugar, and supports cholesterol management. Fiber is found in whole grains, fruits, vegetables, and legumes.

Why Carbohydrates Are Not Considered Essential

The body requires essential nutrients to survive and function properly—nutrients that must be obtained from the diet because the body cannot synthesize them in sufficient quantities. While carbohydrates serve as a primary energy source, the body can produce glucose through gluconeogenesis—a metabolic pathway that creates glucose from non-carbohydrate sources such as proteins and fats. This ability means that, strictly speaking, the body can function without dietary carbohydrates, relying on protein and fat for energy. However, this does not diminish the importance of carbohydrates in a balanced diet, particularly because of the beneficial roles of fiber and the energy supplied by complex carbohydrates for overall health and well-being.

Recommend Intake

The amount of carbohydrates you should consume daily depends on various personal factors like your age, gender, level of physical activity, and specific health objectives. Generally, the dietary guidelines recommend that 45% to 65% of your total daily calorie intake should come from carbohydrates. For an individual on a 2,000-calorie diet, this amounts to 225 to 325 grams of carbs daily.

When choosing carbohydrates, it's crucial to emphasize the quality:

- Opt for complex carbohydrates such as those in whole grains, fruits, vegetables, and beans, which are rich in fiber and essential nutrients.
- Reduce intake of simple sugars and refined carbs found in sugary beverages, desserts, and processed foods to avoid rapid blood sugar spikes and potential health issues.

Tailoring your carb intake to fit your unique needs is best done with guidance from a health professional or dietitian, ensuring your diet effectively supports your health and wellness goals.

Carbohydrate Sources:

Complex Carbohydrates (Good Sources):

- Whole grains (e.g., brown rice, quinoa, oats)
- Legumes (e.g., lentils, chickpeas, black beans)
- Vegetables (e.g., broccoli, carrots, leafy greens)
- Fruits (e.g., apples, berries, oranges)

- Tubers (e.g., sweet potatoes, yams)

Simple Carbohydrates (Consume in Moderation):

- Sugary foods (e.g., candy, cookies)
- Refined grains (e.g., white bread, white pasta)
- Sugary drinks (e.g., soda, sweetened beverages)
- Processed snacks (e.g., chips, crackers)

Fiber-Rich Foods:

- Fruits (e.g., pears, avocados, bananas)
- Vegetables (e.g., Brussels sprouts, artichokes)
- Whole grains (e.g., barley, bran flakes)
- Legumes (e.g., beans, lentils)
- Nuts and seeds (e.g., almonds, chia seeds)

Incorporating a variety of complex carbohydrates and fiber-rich foods into your diet can help ensure a balanced intake of nutrients, while simple carbohydrates should be limited to maintain overall health.

Carb Cycling: An Overview

Carb cycling is a dietary approach where you alternate between high-carb and low-carb days throughout the week. The strategy aims to match the body's need for carbohydrates based on daily activity levels, potentially maximizing benergy use for workouts, aiding in weight management, and improving muscle recovery. Athletes and bodybuilders often use it, but it can be adapted by anyone looking to optimize their carbohydrate intake for health or fitness goals.

How Carb Cycling Works:

- High-Carb Days: Typically coincide with heavy workout days, providing ample energy for high-intensity exercise and supporting muscle growth and recovery.
- Low-Carb Days: Align with rest or light activity days, helping to manage calorie intake and potentially encourage fat burning.

Benefits of Carb Cycling:

- Flexibility in diet planning.
- Can support both weight loss and muscle gain goals.
- May help regulate blood sugar levels and improve insulin sensitivity.

Implementing Carb Cycling:

- Plan Your Week: Align high-carb days with your most intense training sessions and low-carb days with rest or light activity days.
- Choose Quality Carbs: On high-carb days, focus on complex carbohydrates like whole grains, fruits, and vegetables. On low-carb days, still include non-starchy vegetables for fiber and nutrients.
- Monitor Your Body's Response: Adjust your carb cycling plan based on your energy levels, workout performance, and progress toward your goals.

Fun Facts:

- *Historical Diets: The varying diet based on daily activity isn't new. Ancient hunter-gatherers' diets naturally cycled based on seasonal availability and daily exertion levels.*
- *Not Just for Weight Loss: While often associated with fat loss, carb cycling*

can also be a powerful tool for building muscle, especially when high-carb days support heavy lifting sessions.

- *Adaptable for Everyone: Carb cycling doesn't require strict adherence to specific carb counts, making it a flexible approach that can suit various dietary preferences and lifestyle needs.*

Carb cycling offers an adaptable approach to carbohydrate intake, allowing for dietary variation that aligns with your fitness routine and goals. Whether you're looking to lose fat, build muscle, or simply enhance your diet's effectiveness, carb cycling can be a strategic tool to consider. Remember, as with any dietary strategy, individual results may vary, and it's important to listen to your body and adjust as needed.

Weekly Carb Cycling Plan Example:

- Monday (High-Carb Day): Align with a heavy strength training session. Aim for 50-60% of your daily calories from carbohydrates. Focus on complex carbs like sweet potatoes, whole grains, and fruits.
- Tuesday (Low-Carb Day): Schedule a rest day or light activity day. Reduce carbs to 20-30% of your daily calories, emphasizing non-starchy vegetables and lean proteins to fill your plate.
- Wednesday (High-Carb Day): Coincide with another intense workout day, such as sprint intervals or a long-distance run. Follow the same high-carb guidelines as Monday.
- Thursday (Moderate-Carb Day): Use for a moderate workout, like a steady-state cardio session. Carbs can be 40% of your daily calories, balancing between sources like legumes, dairy, and whole fruits.
- Friday (Low-Carb Day): Align with a rest day or a very light workout, such as yoga. Keep carb intake on the lower side, similar to Tuesday.

- Saturday (High-Carb Day): Plan for a high-intensity workout, such as a heavy lifting day or a challenging group fitness class. This is another day to increase carb intake significantly to support energy needs and recovery.
- Sunday (Low-Carb Day): Typically a rest day or active recovery day with light walking or stretching. Carb intake should be minimized, similar to other low-carb days.

Key Points for Carb Cycling:

- Adjust Portions According to Needs: The exact amount of carbs will vary based on your total caloric needs, weight, and fitness goals. It's essential to tailor the plan to your individual requirements.
- Quality of Carbohydrates: On high-carb days, prioritize complex, nutrient-dense carbohydrates. On low-carb days, focus on maintaining adequate fiber intake through vegetables and low-glycemic fruits.
- Protein and Fat Intake: While carb intake varies, protein intake should remain relatively constant to support muscle repair and growth. Fat intake can be adjusted inversely with carb intake to help meet energy needs.

This example of carb cycling is just a template. Individuals may need to adjust their carb-cycling plan based on personal goals, responses, and preferences. Consulting with a nutritionist or dietitian can provide personalized guidance for optimal results.

CONCLUSION

Our exploration of carbohydrates highlights their importance as a primary energy source and their role in a balanced diet. We've differentiated between simple and complex carbohydrates and discussed the significance of fiber. Additionally, we've introduced carb cycling to align carbohydrate intake with energy needs and fitness goals.

Key takeaways include:

- Carbohydrates are necessary for energy and various bodily functions.
- Choosing the correct type of carbohydrates—preferring complex carbs and fiber-rich foods—is crucial for health.
- Carb cycling can be a practical approach for managing carb intake, especially for those with specific performance or body composition goals.

It's essential to tailor carbohydrate consumption to individual needs, focusing on whole foods for optimal health benefits. Understanding and managing your carb intake can support energy levels, promote health, and contribute to achieving dietary goals.

7

HORMONES

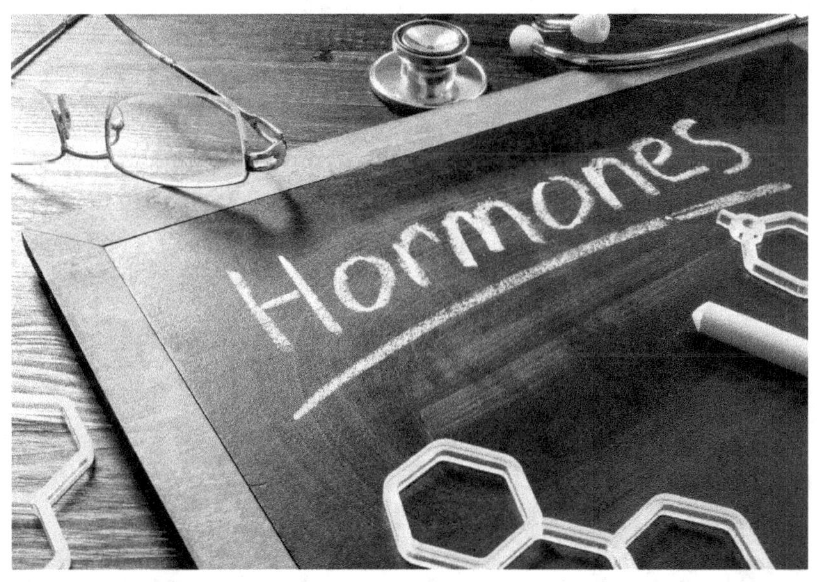

Practical Guide to Diet and Hormonal Health:

Your diet significantly influences your hormonal balance, affecting your overall health. Here's a straightforward look at how certain foods impact hormones and some actionable advice:

- Impact of Sugar on Insulin: Regularly consuming high amounts of sugar can cause your body to become less responsive to insulin, leading to higher blood sugar levels. Practical tip: Adding spices like cinnamon to your meals can naturally help manage blood sugar levels.
- Benefits of Omega-3s: Foods rich in omega-3 fatty acids, like salmon and flaxseeds, help reduce inflammation, facilitating better hormonal communication. Quick fact: Including fish in your diet a few times a week can support hormone health.
- The Role of Protein: Proteins are crucial for hormone production and balance. Incorporating protein sources like Greek yogurt or almonds into your daily diet ensures your body has the necessary building blocks for hormones. Real-life tip: Starting your day with a protein-rich breakfast can help maintain stable energy levels.
- Importance of Hydration for Hormones: Staying well-hydrated aids in cellular function and hormone production. Keeping a water bottle handy and sipping throughout the day can ensure your hormonal system functions smoothly.

Real Examples:

Case Study: Emma: Emma swapped her sugary snacks for healthier options like nuts and added more omega-3-rich foods to her diet. This shift improved her energy and had a visible effect on her skin health.

Case Study: John: After cutting out sugary drinks in favor of lemon-infused sparkling water, John experienced more stable energy levels throughout the day, eliminating the usual afternoon energy dips.

By understanding how your diet affects your hormones, you can make practical changes to improve your health. Minor adjustments, such as reducing sugar intake and increasing omega-3 and protein-rich foods, can significantly impact your hormonal balance and overall well-being.

Testosterone: Its Role in Men and Women

Testosterone, commonly recognized for its role in male health, is crucial for both men and women, influencing various bodily functions and contributing to overall well-being.

Testosterone in Men:

- Primary Male Sex Hormone: Testosterone is pivotal in developing male sexual characteristics, including muscle mass, bone density, and body hair. It also plays a key role in sperm production.
- Health Impacts: Beyond its reproductive functions, testosterone influences mood, energy levels, and cognitive function in men. Optimal levels are essential for cardiovascular health, muscle strength, and preventing osteoporosis.

Testosterone in Women:

- Vital but in Smaller Amounts: Women produce testosterone in their ovaries and adrenal glands, albeit in much lower quantities compared to men. It's essential for ovarian function, bone strength, and libido.
- Balance is Key: In women, a delicate testosterone balance is crucial. Too little can lead to a lack of sexual desire, fatigue, and bone loss, while too much may cause symptoms like excess hair growth and

acne.

Testosterone in Your Body:

- Production and Regulation: Testosterone levels are regulated by the hypothalamus and pituitary gland, signaling the testes in men and ovaries in women to produce the hormone. Levels naturally decline with age in both genders.
- Maintaining Healthy Levels: Diet and lifestyle play significant roles in maintaining healthy testosterone levels. Regular exercise, particularly strength training and HIIT, can boost testosterone production. Nutritional factors, including adequate protein intake and certain minerals like zinc and vitamin D, are also important.

Practical Tips:

- For Men and Women: Engaging in regular physical activity and ensuring a balanced diet rich in nutrients can support optimal testosterone levels. Managing stress through mindfulness or relaxation techniques can also help, as chronic stress may lead to hormonal imbalances.

Understanding the role of testosterone and how it differs in men and women underscores the importance of this hormone in your health. Whether it's supporting sexual health, maintaining muscle mass, or ensuring emotional well-being, testosterone plays a key role across genders. Making informed lifestyle and dietary choices can help manage testosterone levels effectively.

Understanding Cortisol: The Stress Hormone

Cortisol, often dubbed the "stress hormone," is produced by the adrenal glands and plays a crucial role in various bodily functions. It's best known for its involvement in the body's stress response, but its influence extends to metabolism, immune response, and blood pressure regulation.

Key Functions of Cortisol:

- Stress Response: Cortisol is released in response to stress, preparing the body to either fight or flee by increasing glucose in the bloodstream and enhancing the brain's use of glucose.
- Metabolism Regulation: It helps regulate metabolism by supporting the breakdown of fats, proteins, and carbohydrates, providing energy for the body.
- Immune System Modulation: Cortisol has anti-inflammatory effects and can modulate the immune system, suppressing excessive immune reactions.
- Blood Pressure and Heart Function: It supports maintaining blood pressure and cardiovascular function during stressful situations.

Cortisol and Health:

While cortisol is essential for survival, chronic high levels due to prolonged stress can lead to several health issues:

- Weight Gain: High cortisol can increase appetite and signal the body to store fat, particularly in the abdominal area.
- Sleep Problems: It can disrupt sleep patterns, making falling or staying asleep hard.
- Immune Function: Over time, elevated cortisol levels can weaken the immune system, making the body more susceptible to infec-

tions.

- Mood Disorders: Chronic stress and high cortisol can contribute to anxiety, depression, and memory issues.

Managing Cortisol Levels:

- Stress Management: Techniques like meditation, yoga, or deep breathing can reduce stress and lower cortisol levels.
- Regular Exercise: Physical activity, especially aerobic exercises, can help balance cortisol levels, improve mood, and enhance overall health.
- Healthy Diet: A balanced diet with plenty of fruits, vegetables, whole grains, and lean protein can support adrenal function and cortisol regulation.
- Adequate Sleep: Ensuring sufficient, quality sleep each night helps regulate cortisol production and supports recovery and stress management.

Fun Fact:

- *Cortisol Awakening Response (CAR): Cortisol levels naturally peak about 30 minutes after waking in a phenomenon known as the cortisol awakening response, helping to energize the body for the day ahead.*

Cortisol plays a multifaceted role in your health, highlighting the importance of managing stress and adopting a healthy lifestyle to keep cortisol levels in check. By understanding cortisol's impact on the body, individuals can take proactive steps to maintain balance, supporting physical and mental well-being.

Conclusion

This chapter highlights the importance of key hormones like testosterone and cortisol in health management. Testosterone plays a critical role in sexual function, muscle growth, and mood for both genders. Cortisol, the stress hormone, affects metabolism, the immune system, and stress responses. Imbalanced levels of these hormones can lead to various issues, including weight changes, sleep disturbances, and mood fluctuations. Maintaining hormonal balance involves regular exercise, effective stress management, a nutritious diet, and sufficient sleep. It's crucial to manage these hormones properly for optimal health.

8

HYDRATION

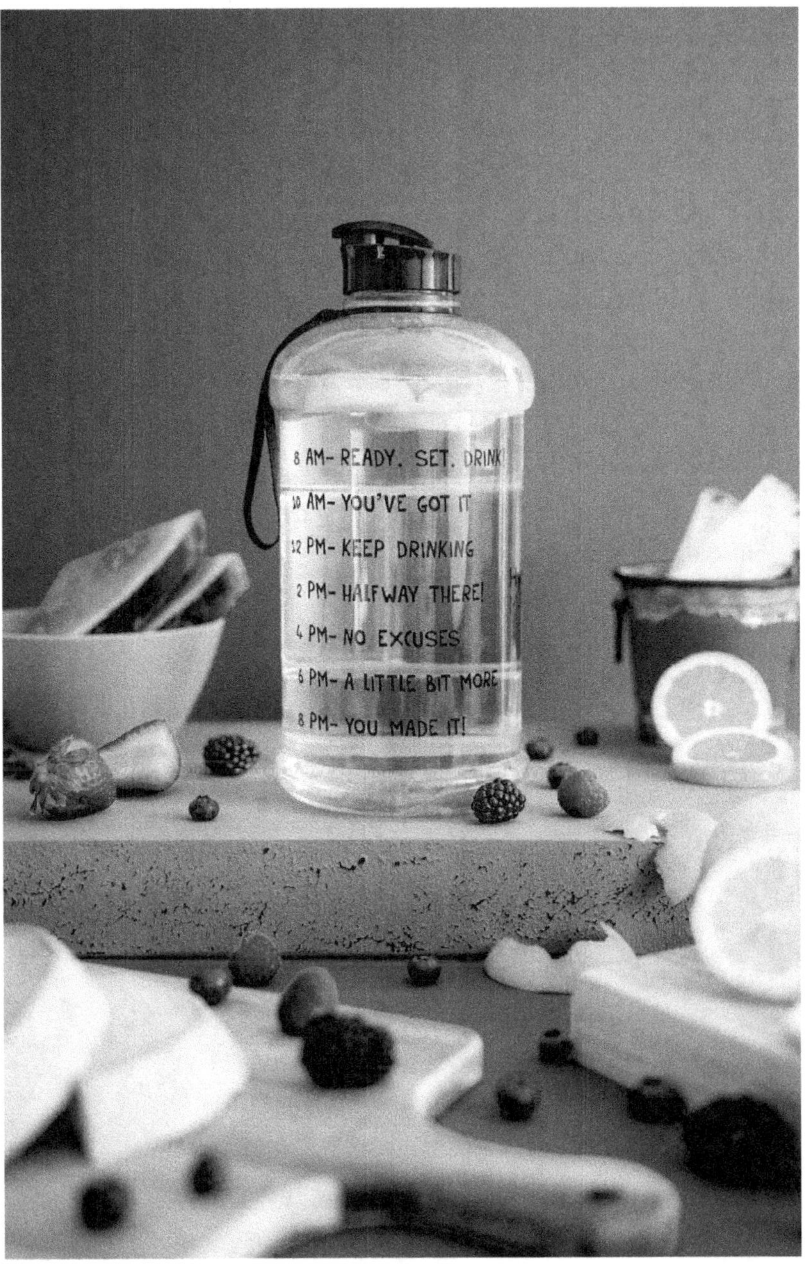
8 AM- READY. SET. DRINK
10 AM- YOU'VE GOT IT
12 PM- KEEP DRINKING
2 PM- HALFWAY THERE!
4 PM- NO EXCUSES
6 PM- A LITTLE BIT MORE
8 PM- YOU MADE IT!

Hydration: The Cornerstone of Wellness

Hydration isn't just about drinking water; it's a critical component of health, influencing everything from physical performance to cognitive function. Let's break down the essentials of hydration, including how our bodies handle water, the impact of dehydration, and how to stay properly hydrated, especially when active.

How Our Bodies Manage Water

- Water Absorption: The small intestine plays a key role in absorbing water, where electrolytes like sodium and potassium help pull water into the body's cells.
- Water Loss: Daily activities see us losing water through sweat, urine, and even breath. Fun fact: An average person loses about 1 to 1.5 liters of water daily just through urine!

The Downside of Not Drinking Enough

Dehydration can sneak up on us, impacting more than just our thirst levels. It can lead to:

- Diminished strength and stamina
- Brain fog and concentration difficulties
- Constipation and digestive discomfort
- Potential kidney issues over time

Symptoms to watch for include persistent thirst, dry skin, dizziness, and more amber urine than usual.

Tailoring Hydration to Activity Levels

Engaging in exercise, especially in warm conditions, ups our water loss, making it crucial to adjust our fluid intake. Here are some guidelines:

- Pre-Workout: Drink about 500ml (17 ounces) of water a couple of hours before hitting the gym to ensure you're starting well-hydrated.
- Mid-Workout Hydration: Losing just 2% of your body weight in fluid can reduce performance, so keep sipping water every 15 minutes or so during exercise.
- Post-Workout: For every pound of weight lost during your workout, aim to drink 24 ounces of water to rehydrate.

Practical Hydration Tips with a Twist

- Infuse Your Water: Make hydration more enjoyable by infusing water with fruits like lemon, berries, or cucumber for a flavor boost.
- Eat Your Water: Yes, you can eat your water! Fruits and vegetables like watermelon, cucumber, and oranges are packed with water and electrolytes.
- Tech to the Rescue: Use a hydration app to track your water intake and get daily reminders to drink.

Fun Fact: *Did you know that cucumbers are 96% water, making them a perfect snack for hydration?*

Maintaining hydration is essential for health, significantly impacting physical and mental performance. By understanding how to manage hydration, especially in relation to activity effectively, you can support your body's needs, ensuring you stay at the top of your game.

9

SUPPLEMENTS and DIETING METHOD

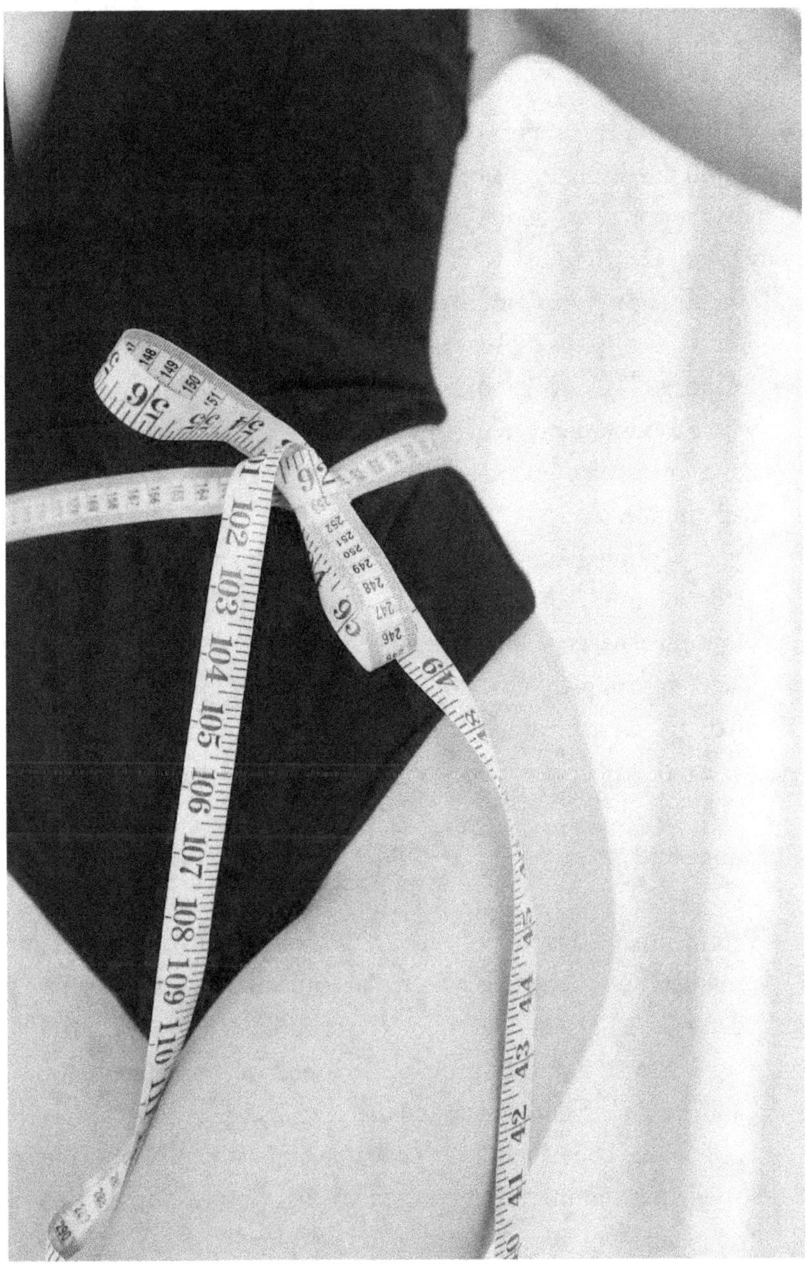

Supplements: Enhancing Your Nutritional Intake

Supplements serve as an adjunct to a balanced diet, designed to fill nutritional gaps or bolster the intake of key nutrients that support the body's functions, including the immune system and overall body balance.

Key Points on Supplements:

- Purpose: They are intended to supplement the diet, not replace whole foods. Supplements can provide vitamins, minerals, antioxidants, and other essential nutrients that might be lacking in your daily intake.
- Types: Common supplements include multivitamins, omega-3 fatty acids, vitamin D, probiotics, and protein powders, each targeting different aspects of health and wellness.
- Choosing Supplements: Look for products from reputable manufacturers. Certifications or third-party testing can offer assurance of quality and purity.

Guidance and Safety:

- Professional Consultation: It's crucial to consult with healthcare providers before starting any supplement regimen, especially if you have existing health conditions or are taking medication. Healthcare professionals can provide personalized recommendations based on your health needs and dietary habits.
- Supporting Your Health Goals: Supplements siments can play a role in supporting immune function, enhancing physical performance, and promoting overall health, but they should be part of a comprehensive approach that includes a nutritious diet and regular exercise.

Practical Tip:

- Informed Choices: Utilize resources like registered dietitians or pharmacists to gain insights into which supplements might benefit you. They can help you understand the appropriate dosages and the best time of day to take supplements for optimal absorption and effectiveness.

It's essential to navigate the world of supplements with informed caution, ensuring that any additions to your diet support rather than compromise your health. Supplements can be a valuable tool in your wellness arsenal when used appropriately and under professional guidance

Key Points on Supplements:

- Purpose:
- Intended to supplement, not replace, a nutritious diet.
- Provide essential nutrients that may be lacking.
- Types:
- Multivitamins for broad nutritional coverage.
- Specific supplements targeting unique health needs.

Essential and Recommended Supplements:

- Fish Oil:
- Rich in omega-3 fatty acids.
- Supports heart health and cognitive function.
- Vitamin D:
- Essential for bone health and immune function.
- Many individuals are deficient, especially in areas with less sunlight.
- Magnesium:

- Crucial for muscle function and energy production.
- Can aid in sleep and stress management.
- Vitamin C:
- Supports immune system health.
- Important for skin and tissue repair.
- BCAAs (Branched-Chain Amino Acids):
- Support muscle recovery and growth.
- Can reduce exercise fatigue.

Guidance and Safety:

- Professional Consultation: Always consult healthcare professionals to tailor supplement use to your individual health needs.
- Choosing Supplements:
- Opt for quality brands with third-party testing.
- Be wary of supplements with exaggerated claims.

Practical Tip:

- Informed Choices: Leverage advice from registered dietitians or healthcare providers to understand which supplements and dosages are best for you.

Navigating supplement use requires informed decisions and professional guidance to ensure they effectively support your health and nutritional goals. Supplements like fish oil, vitamin D, magnesium, vitamin C, and BCAAs can offer significant health benefits when used appropriately as part of a well-rounded wellness strategy.

Evaluating Popular Dieting Methods: Pros and Cons

Dieting strategies vary widely, each with its advantages and drawbacks. Understanding these can help you choose the most suitable approach for your health and wellness goals.

Clean Eating

- Pros:
- Promotes overall health with a focus on whole foods.
- Can lead to sustainable weight management.
- Reduces intake of processed foods and added sugars.
- Cons:
- May be time-consuming due to meal preparation.
- Potentially more expensive depending on food choices

Macro Approach (Flexible Dieting)

- Pros:
- Offers flexibility in food choices while meeting nutritional goals.
- Can be tailored to various objectives, such as weight loss or muscle gain.
- Encourages awareness of macronutrient balance and portion sizes.
- Cons:
- Requires tracking and calculating macros, which can be tedious.
- Might lead to an overemphasis on numbers rather than food quality.

Fasting (Time-Restricted Eating)

- Pros:
- Simplifies dieting by focusing on meal timing rather than calorie counting.
- May improve metabolic health and increase fat loss.
- Can enhance discipline and reduce overall calorie intake.

- Cons:
- Potential for overeating during eating windows.
- May cause fatigue or irritability during fasting periods.
- Not suitable for everyone, especially those with certain health conditions.

Keto (Low-Carb/High-Fat)

- Pros:
- Can lead to significant weight loss and improved blood sugar control.
- May reduce appetite, leading to a natural decrease in calorie intake.
- Supports mental clarity and energy levels for some individuals.
- Cons:
- Restrictive and can be difficult to maintain long-term.
- May cause initial side effects, such as the "keto flu."
- Potential nutrient deficiencies if not properly planned.

Meal Replacements (Shakes and Pre-packaged Meals)

- Pros:
- Convenient and easy to manage, especially for those with a busy lifestyle.
- Controlled portions can aid in weight loss.
- Nutritionally balanced options ensure essential nutrient intake.
- Cons:
- Lack of variety may lead to boredom and potential nutrient imbalances.
- Some products may be high in sugars and additives.
- Less satisfying than whole foods, potentially leading to snacking.

Choosing a dieting method involves weighing these pros and cons against your personal health goals, lifestyle, and preferences. It's often beneficial to consult with a healthcare professional or nutritionist to tailor a plan that suits your needs and ensures a balanced, nutritious diet.

Conclusion

This chapter focused on the role of dietary supplements and different dieting techniques in supporting health and nutrition goals. Supplements are useful for filling in nutritional gaps, offering a convenient source of vitamins, minerals, and other nutrients that you might not get enough of from food alone. It's important to select trusted brands and seek advice from healthcare professionals to tailor supplement choices to your specific needs.

Additionally, we examined several dieting methods, including clean eating, macro tracking, intermittent fasting, the ketogenic diet, and meal replacement strategies. Each method has its advantages, whether aiding in weight loss, improving metabolic health, or simplifying meal planning. However, they also come with considerations such as sustainability, ease of adherence, and potential nutritional completeness.

Choosing the right supplements and dieting approach requires a clear understanding of your health objectives and lifestyle preferences. Consulting with a nutritionist or a healthcare provider can help customize your diet plan to ensure it's effective, sustainable, and aligned with your overall health goals.

10

MINDSET

ATTITUDE
BEHAVIOUR
MINDSET
ACTION
SOLUTION
PERFORMANCE
RESULTS

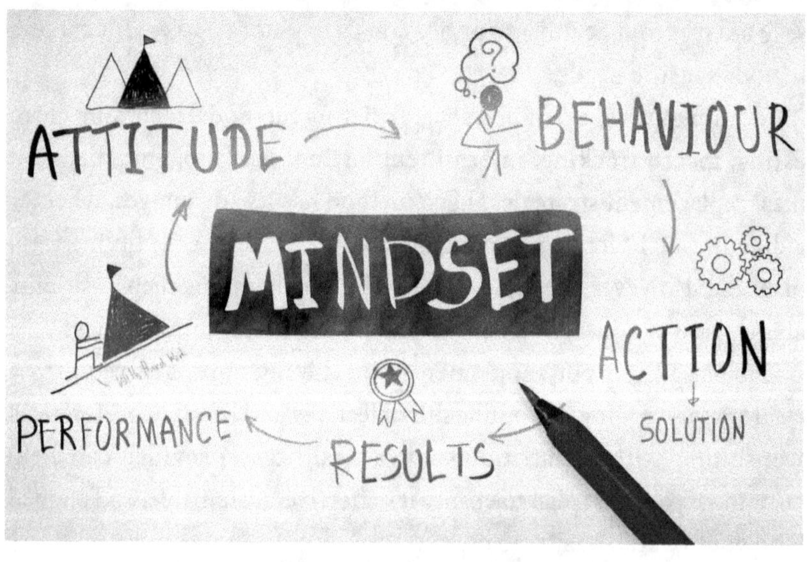

Mindset: The Foundation of Wellness

The power of a good mindset and positive self-talk cannot be overstated when it comes to achieving health and wellness goals. Mindset refers to the established set of attitudes held by someone, and it plays a pivotal role in how we approach our daily lives, including our health and fitness journeys.

The Power of a Good Mindset:

- Influences Behavior: A positive mindset motivates us to adopt healthy behaviors and persist through challenges. Believing in the possibility of change encourages consistent effort toward goals.
- Shapes Perception: Our mindset heavily influences how we perceive challenges and setbacks. Viewing difficulties as opportunities for growth rather than insurmountable obstacles can lead to greater resilience and success.
- Impacts Outcomes: Studies have shown that individuals with a positive outlook are more likely to achieve their health and fitness goals. This positivity breeds further success, creating a virtuous cycle of improvement.

The Role of Positive Self-Talk:

- Boosts Confidence: Regularly affirming your abilities and worth helps build self-confidence, which is crucial for overcoming barriers to health and fitness.
- Reduces Stress: Positive self-talk can help reframe stressful situations, reducing stress's psychological and physiological impact on the body.
- Enhances Performance: Athletes who engage in positive self-talk are shown to perform better and have greater endurance, highlight-

ing the direct link between mindset and physical performance.

Cultivating a Positive Mindset:

- Practice Gratitude: Regularly acknowledging what you're thankful for can shift focus from what's lacking to what's abundant, fostering a positive outlook.
- Set Realistic Goals: Achievable goals reinforce a sense of accomplishment and competence, fueling positive thoughts and actions.
- Surround Yourself with Positivity: The company you keep can influence your mindset. Engage with supportive, optimistic individuals who encourage your wellness journey.

A positive mindset and self-talk are essential tools in the pursuit of health and wellness. They empower us to face challenges with resilience, embrace personal growth, and achieve our goals with confidence. Cultivating these mental habits lays the foundation for lasting change and a fulfilling life.

Here are some engaging facts about the impact of mindset on our health and daily life:

- Brain Adaptability: Your brain can change structure and function based on your thoughts, thanks to a phenomenon called neuroplasticity. Adopting a positive mindset feels good and can create lasting positive changes in your brain.
- The Power of Belief: The placebo effect showcases how strong belief in a treatment, even if it's just a sugar pill, can lead to real health improvements. It highlights how expectations can significantly influence our physical health.
- Longevity and Optimism: Research indicates that optimists tend

to live longer and enjoy better health, including a reduced risk of heart disease. A sunny outlook on life is associated with healthier habits and stress management.

- Forced Smiles Work Wonders: Simply smiling can signal to your brain that you're happy, leading to actual feelings of joy. This is a testament to the close link between our facial expressions and our emotions.
- Gratitude for Better Sleep: The practice of jotting down what you're thankful for each night can lead to improved sleep quality. Focusing on positive aspects of your life helps ease the mind into a more restful state.
- Never-Ending Learning: Continually challenging yourself to learn new things not only enriches your life but also strengthens your brain, reinforcing the idea that growth and development continue throughout life.
- Meditation's Lasting Effects: Regular meditation practice can literally thicken areas of the brain responsible for attention and emotion regulation. This demonstrates that mindfulness can have tangible, beneficial changes in brain structure.

These intriguing facts emphasize the powerful role of mindset in shaping our experience of the world, influencing everything from our physical health to our capacity for happiness and learning. Cultivating a positive, growth-oriented mindset is a key component of living a fulfilled and healthy life.

To cultivate a healthy mindset, consider incorporating these ten daily practices:

- Practice Gratitude: Start or end your day by listing three things you're grateful for to foster positivity.

- Set Intentions for the Day: Each morning, set clear, positive intentions for what you wish to achieve.
- Engage in Physical Activity: Regular exercise boosts mood and reduces stress, contributing to a positive outlook.
- Mindful Meditation: Dedicate a few minutes to mindfulness or meditation to reduce stress and enhance focus.
- Positive Affirmations: Use affirmations to reinforce self-esteem and confidence throughout the day.
- Limit Social Media: Reduce time on social media to avoid comparison and information overload.
- Nourish Your Body: Eat balanced, nutritious meals to fuel both body and mind.
- Connect with Loved Ones: Spend quality time with friends or family to strengthen emotional support.
- Learn Something New: Challenge your brain by learning a new skill or hobby, promoting growth and satisfaction.
- Reflect and Adjust: End your day by reflecting on what went well and how you can improve, turning challenges into opportunities for growth.

Conclusion

Wrapping up our discussion on mindset, we've seen how crucial a positive outlook is for overall health and happiness. Implementing daily practices such as expressing gratitude, setting goals, staying active, and practicing mindfulness can significantly contribute to a healthier mindset. Incorporating positive affirmations, reducing social media usage, eating well, connecting with others, learning new things, and reflecting on your day are practical steps that improve mental and emotional well-being.

These strategies help build a positive mindset and have tangible benefits for physical health, enhancing relationships, and effectively dealing with life's ups and downs. By actively engaging in these practices, you take control of your mental health, laying a strong foundation for a balanced and satisfying life. This chapter highlights the importance of a proactive approach to cultivating a positive mindset, offering readers actionable steps to make meaningful changes in their outlook and life.

11

CONCLUSION

CONCLUSION

In the final pages of this book, I reflect on the journey of sharing what has truly been a labor of love for me. My ultimate goal has always been to make a difference, even if it's just for one person, to help them live their best life.

In our fast-paced, often overwhelming world, getting lost in the endless to-dos is easy. Whether we're parents, siblings, coworkers, or friends, the demands on our time and energy can be relentless. But here's the thing—self-care isn't just a buzzword; it's a necessity. It's vital to pause, breathe, and take that moment for yourself, whether it's a peaceful walk, a rejuvenating run, or indulging in an hour-long massage. Self-care is the key to resilience and vitality.

Growing up, a piece of wisdom my mother imparted to me was the importance of helping oneself to be capable of helping others. This advice rings especially true in an era where anxiety and depression are on the rise. Paying attention to the signs our bodies and minds give us, nourishing ourselves with good food, engaging in meaningful movement, and living with intention is foundational to well-being.

"10 Hard Truths":

- You are 100% responsible for your own happiness.
- Your health is your true wealth.
- You can't control most things except how you respond.
- Nothing worth having comes easy.
- Failure is a prerequisite for success.
- Not everyone is going to like you.
- To help others, you must first take care of yourself.
- Actions speak louder than words.
- Vulnerability and asking for help are strengths.
- Life is precious, and so are you.

These truths serve as a guiding light, reminding us of the fundamental principles that lead to a fulfilling and meaningful life. As this book comes to a close, I hope it ignites a spark within you to embrace these lessons, prioritize your well-being, and remember—that the power to shape your life and happiness lies within you. Thank you for joining me on this journey. Here's to living a life that's good for ourselves and enriches those around us.

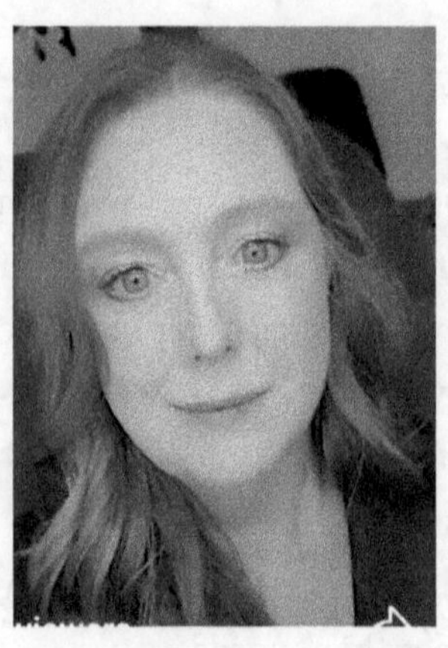

About the Author

I am a wife to my Husband and best friend. Together, we have 4 exceptional children. I am obsessed with my dogs. I have a French pug and a Vizsla. We spend a lot of time exploring the outdoors, walking, hiking, and camping, and when not outdoors, we enjoy the Gym, Spa treatments, and relaxation. It is pivotal for our Well-being. I have always enjoyed and thrived on Health and Wellness, and I believe in nourishing our minds and bodies. My passion has always been to help others understand and navigate their nutrition, well-being, and Happiness.

www.ingramcontent.com/pod-product-compliance
Lightning Source LLC
Chambersburg PA
CBHW050839260726

48660CB00006B/2332